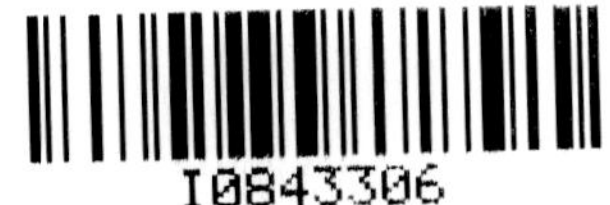# This notebook belongs to:

....

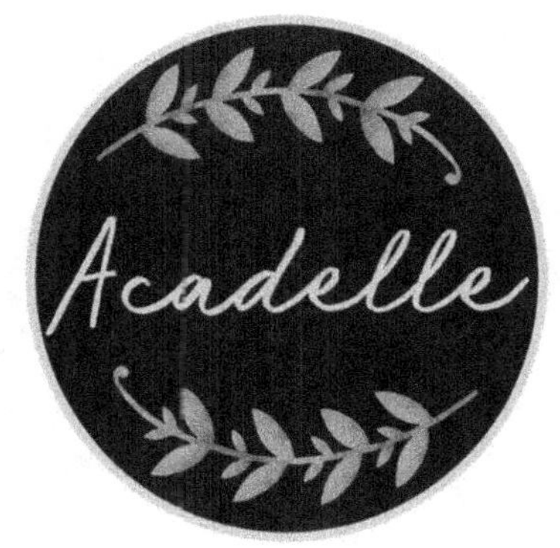

Visit us at www.acadelle.com for more notebooks, planners and other awesome vegan goodies.

Follow us on Facebook:
facebook.com/acadelle

Eat More Hole Foods